Alkaline  Paleo

How to Combine Alkaline Diet and Paleo Diet for Wellness, Weight Loss, and Vibrant Health!

By Elena Garcia and James Adler
aka the Marriage of Alkaline and Paleo

Table of Contents

Introduction

Would you like to improve your overall health, detox your body on a daily basis, experience endless amounts of energy, lose weight, rev up your sex drive, and boost your mental capacity? Sure, we all would. Yet, most people do not know that you can have all of this simply by changing what you eat.

The good news is that with this book, you will be able to prepare interesting delicious, mouthwatering meals to revolutionize your health and life. When it comes to "dieting", it's not only about weight loss. It's about deep personal transformation and realizing how much you can actually achieve if you get committed to it.

No longer will you have to look for the newest energy drink, supplement, pill, or workout plan that will bring health and wellness. Your search stops here. Slow the process of aging, rid yourself of digestive issues and allergies, and feel better than you ever have before! At the same time, we would like to let you know that there will be no starvation involved. We propose a healthy and balanced diet that is also delicious and will satisfy your taste buds.

WHO ARE WE AND WHY WE WROTE THIS BOOK

We are Elena(Ela) and James, a married couple who found out that through the combination of two of the best dietary plans (we were each a fan of different ones), the marriage of Paleo and Alkaline, we could have everything we have ever wanted or needed in order to mentally and physically function at our finest!! We wanted to share our combined efforts with everyone, which is why we put together this book. There is both a female as well as a male point of view.

We have outlined the basics of our combined efforts, providing you with an easy to understand breakdown of Alkaline Paleo nutrition. Included are shopping lists and recipes that will not only provide you with delicious meals, they will inevitably change your life forever! Put together these meals and provide your body and mind with what they need to allow you to successfully live a healthy, energized lifestyle today. It's easy, fun and exciting. There is no need to survive entirely on greens, we are fans of balance and this is what we want to teach you.

The book you are reading now is our practical vision of how you can combine Alkaline-Paleo diets and create something that works for you. In order to be successful, you should be enjoying your process of transformation. We encourage you to do what we did- experiment and come up with your plan that is exciting and full of nutrients. This book is not strictly Alkaline, we believe that it's all about balance. We have seen way too many of our friends fail with their wellness and weight loss goals because they were trying to be perfect and thought that it was all about eating 100% green alkaline foods. This may be a good idea for an occasional detox plan conducted with an experienced nutritionist, but we personally do not recommended it as an everyday eating plan. We try to be as transparent as possible and simply tell you what we do. Take what you like and reject the rest. We encourage you to take notes as you read, in case you have any questions, suggestions and doubts, simply email us at:

elenajamesbooks@gmail.com

Our mission is to make things as easy and simple as possible- no fluff. There is no need to devour dozens of advanced nutrition books to be healthy. If you are a busy parent, like we both are, we understand that it can be pretty challenging to eat healthy and keep it tasty at the same time. This is why we came up with an idea of writing a practical dieting book that is full of tips and recipes that you can implement straight away and see results. We suggest you start applying as soon as possible- you will be blown away by the results. Healthy eating is actually easy and fun!

Welcome Gift

Free Complimentary eBook

As a small token of appreciation to you for taking an interest in our work, we have included a free bonus gift which you can claim below.

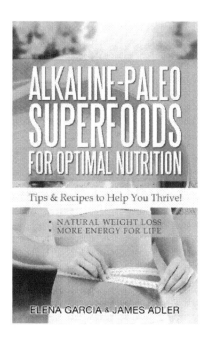

Download link:

www.bitly.com/alkapaleofree

Problems with your download?

Contact us: elenajamesbooks@gmail.com

We will make sure you receive your free eBook as promised.

Chapter 1: Alkalize with an Ancient Twist

By combining two strange sounding, different nutritional lifestyles, we were able to come up with a single dietary plan that is the perfect fit for two equally different and strange people! If it works for us, it can work for you. The key is in the fact that both of these lifestyles were created to help the body function the way that it was designed to. They are set up in a manner that allows them to work *with* the body, instead of fighting to keep it inline. Mixing these blueprint-like nutritional guidelines will allow you to be in spectacular physical and mental health for the rest of your life!

Alkaline: Elena's strong point

The object of eating an alkaline diet is not what it sounds like it might be. There is no battery-eating involved. The objective is to alkalize your body by eating foods and drinking liquids that will encourage a balanced pH environment. The blood's pH is designed to run effectively at 7.35 A "normal," modern diet is full of foods and substances that, when digested, have an acidic effect on the system, causing many problems. Many unwanted health issues can be related to:

- Heart disease

- Allergies

- Gastro-intestinal issues

- Chronic inflammation

- Respiratory problems

- Obesity

- Arthritis

- Skin ailments

- Immune system function

- Hair Loss

- Sexual Dysfunctions

- Muscular, reproductive, excretory, and nervous system malfunctions

In order to get your pH back on track and in balance, it is recommended that we focus on eating 70- 80 percent alkaline forming food. The other 20-30 percent is allowed to be acid-forming (where we decided to apply our "Paleo meat," more on that later). The acid-forming foods should be of course as healthy as possible, I suggest you avoid/eliminate processed foods. The alkaline foods you will need to focus on are mainly vegetables; some non-sugary fruits are allowable (you can keep all kinds of fruits in your acidic 20-30% of your diet).

This was actually easy for me to do (Elena). I enjoyed a vegan diet for most of my adult life and already had a taste for high alkaline foods. Hydration is also a big part of alkalizing the body and I would normally drink so much water that it would make some people balk. James always thought one day I would float away! The first thing I do in the morning is...I .drink a few glasses of alkaline water and I add some green powders. I also like to squeeze in some fresh lemon juice. I usually drink about 1 liter of good quality alkaline water first thing in the morning. It's excellent for digestion!

I believe that alkaline supplements are also extremely important; however the first thing you should focus on is consuming more fresh, alkaline foods. Supplements won't do miracles if you still cheat and stick to your old, unhealthy habits.

Generally we stick to green and root veggies, some fruits, and seeds/nuts. While animal meats and eggs make up most of the other 30-20%. We all do green juice fast about once or twice a year. We also do at least one raw food weekend a month. This is when we give our bodies and digestive tracks some really well-deserved rest. James finds it hard as he loves his meat. But after each cleanse he feels so good that he is utterly grateful I convinced him to join me in this amazing process of detoxification.

Alkaline vs. Acidic?

Sounds like the title fight for a light weight boxing match. In reality it is a fight, a fight for the pH balance of your body. pH levels are basically the measure of how acidic a liquid is. Our bodies function optimally when our blood is at about 7.35 ph. which is slightly alkaline.

Before we dive into complicated pH discussions, here is one thing to understand:

14

-The alkaline <u>diet is not about changing or "raising" your pH</u>. This is where many alkaline guides go wrong. You see, our body is smart enough to self-regulate our pH for us. Unfortunately, when you constantly bombard your body with acid-forming foods (for example processed foods, fast food, alcohol, sugar, and even too much meat) you torture your body with an incredible stress. Why? Well because it has to work harder to maintain that optimal pH...

Here's simple example...

Imagine you immerse yourself in a bath filled with ice. You say, but hey, my body can self-regulate its optimal temperature, right? And yes, it can. But it will eventually collapse and you will get ill. The same happens with nutrition and our blood's pH. You can spend years indulging in toxic, processed, acid-forming foods that only deprive your body of its vital nutrients, saying: "But hey, my body will self-regulate its optimal blood pH".

And again, it will...but sooner or later it will give up and manifest a disease. It will accumulate fat as its natural defense function to protect your body from over-acidity. We don't wanna end up there, right?

So, to sum up- the alkaline diet is a natural, holistic system, a nutritional lifestyle that advocates consumption of fresh, unprocessed foods that are rich in nutrients. These are called alkaline foods and they help your body stimulate its optimal healing functions. Yes! A healthy body needs nutrients and fresh fruits and vegetables are great for that.

The problem is that nowadays, most diets are filled with acid-forming foods that eventually make it hard for the body to regulate its optimal, healthy blood pH and artificial sweeteners do the same. Acidosis is very common in this day and age thanks to things we drink as well: coffee, alcohol, and sodas all have an acidic effect on our bodies. Not to mention the chemicals many people take in through things like smoking and drugs (even prescription drugs have this effect).

There are many ways that you could become acidic. Eating acid forming foods, stress, taking in too many toxins, and bodily processes all cause acidity in the body. Our internal systems try to balance themselves out and bring pH up with the help of alkaline minerals that we can ingest through our diet. If we do not take in a higher percentage of alkaline than acidic foods, we can become too acidic.

When you are acidic, it makes every process that your body normally does much more difficult or impossible for it to accomplish. We cannot absorb the beneficial nutrients we need from our food properly. Our cells are not able to produce energy efficiently. Our bodies are not able to fix damaged cells properly. We will not be able to detoxify properly. Fatigue and illness will drag you down.

Changing your diet to one that is full of alkaline foods is one of the easiest and best things you can do for your overall health. We were so ecstatic that we did! If you are acidic, as we were, you should change your diet immediately. **You should aim to intake 70-80 percent alkaline-forming foods. Sounds pretty easy, right?**

What are alkaline foods? Is it about their pH?

No, luckily it's much, much easier. We don't care about the food's pH in its natural form…All we care about is the effect that the food has on the body after it has been consumed and metabolized. For example, lemons, grapefruits and limes are considered alkaline-forming foods.

What? Elena? James! Are you out of your mind? Everyone knows lemons are acidic…

Well, let us repeat again. Lemons are acidic as far as their taste and ph. in their natural state are concerned. But, they are full of alkaline minerals and low in sugar which makes them alkaline-forming foods.

At the same time, oranges contain more sugar which makes them less alkaline-forming.

Let us repeat:

Some charts determine acidity or alkalinity of the food before it is consumed & others (like the ones we follow and recommend) are more interested in the effect the food has on the body after it has been consumed.

It's really that simple!

As a general rule, alkaline foods are:
-rich in minerals and vitamins
-fresh, not packaged
-not fermented
-low in sugar (all kinds of sugar are acid-forming)
-plant-based
-mostly raw or slightly cooked
-caffeine-free
-chemical-free
-provide hydration
-naturally gluten-free

So let's have a look at the food lists. We think that after our intro it will be easier for you to understand the difference between alkaline and acid forming foods, even without looking at the charts...

One more thing- we base our food lists on Doctor Young's latest research.

We know it is quite confusing to see so many different charts online. We have been there.

The reason why so many other charts show such disparity is because they base their classifications on the readings for the so called PRAL which stands for Potential Renal Acid Load research. Unfortunately, this is not a reliable source of practical information for us.

Why?

Well PRAL tests burn the food at an extreme temperature and then take a read of the 'ash' that is left behind and what it's pH is.

While this will give a read of its alkalinity from the mineral content of the food, by burning it at such a high temperature they also burn away sugar. And sugar is very acid-forming... That is why on some charts high sugar fruits are listed as super alkaline. Now we are not saying that fruits are bad for you, most fruits are neutral or mildly alkaline forming and great as a natural snack or a part of a balanced diet. But they are not as alkalizing as most veggies are.

Some charts determine acidity or alkalinity on the food before it is consumed & others like the ones we list below, are more interested in the effect the food has on the body after it has been consumed.

ALKALIZING VEGETABLES

Asparagus

Broccoli

Chili

Pepper

Zucchini

Dandelion

Snowpeas

Green Beans

String Beans

Runner Beans

Spinach

Kale

Wakame

Kelp

Collards

Chives

Endive

Chard

Cabbage

Sweet Potato

Mint

Ginger

Coriander

Basil

Brussels Sprouts

Cauliflower

Carrot

Beetroot

Eggplant

Garlic

Onion

Parsley

Celery

Cucumber

Watercress

Lettuce

Peas

Broad Beans

New Potato

Pumpkin

Radish

ALKALIZING FRUITS

Avocado

Tomato

Lemon

Lime

Grapefruit

Fresh Coconut

Pomegranate

ALKALIZING PROTEIN

Almonds,

Chestnuts,

Protein Powders (we love hemp)

ALKALINE OILS

Avocado Oil

Coconut Oil

Flax Oil

Udo's Oil

Olive Oil

Other:

Alkaline Water

Fresh Almond Milk

Herbal Tea

ALKALINE SUPERFOODS:

Wheatgrass

Barley Grass

Kamut Grass

Dog Grass

Shave Grass

Oat Grass

Soy Sprouts

Alfalfa Sprouts

Amaranth Sprouts

Broccoli Sprouts

ALKALIZING SWEETENERS
-Stevia (natural)

ALKALIZING SPICES & SEASONINGS
-Chili Peppers,

-Cinnamon,

-Curry,

-Ginger,

-Herbs,

-Sea Salt,

ALKALIZING NUTS AND SEEDS
Almonds

Coconut

Flax Seeds

Pumpkin Seeds

Sesame Seeds

Sunflower Seeds

ACID SWEETENERS

Carob, Corn Syrup, Sugar

ACID BEVERAGES

Alcohol, Coffee, Soda

ACID TOXINS AND DRUGS

All drugs, Weed killers, Insecticides, Tobacco

ACID MEAT:

Bacon

Beef

Clams

Corned Beef

Eggs

Lamb

Lobster

Mussels

Organ Meats

Venison

Fish

Oyster

Pork

Rabbit

Sausage

Scallops

Shellfish

Shrimp

Tuna

Turkey

Veal

MIDLY ACID-FORMING/NEUTRAL FRUITS:

Apple

Apricot

Currants

Dates

Grapes

Mango

Peach

Pear

Prunes

Raisins

Raspberries

Strawberries

Tropical Fruits

Cantaloupe

Cranberries

Currants

Honeydew Melon

Orange

Pineapple

Plum

ACID FORMING DAIRY AND EGGS

Butter

Cheese

Milk

Whey

Yogurt

Cottage Cheese

Ice Cream

Sour Cream

Soy Cheese

Eggs

ACID FORMING OILS

Cooked Oil

Solid Oil (Margarine)

Oil Exposed to Heat,

Light or Air

ACID FORMING DRINKS

Alcohol

Black Tea

Coffee

Carbonated Water

Pasteurized Juice

Cocoa

Energy Drinks

Sports Drinks

Colas

Tap Water

Milk

Green Tea

Decaffeinated Drinks

Flavoured Water

ACID-FORMING SAUCES

Mayonnaise

Ketchup

Mustard

Soy Sauce

Pickles

Vinegar

Tabasco

Tamari

Wasabi

Other ACID-FORMING FOODS:

Mushrooms

Miso

White Breads, Pastas,

Rice & Noodles

Chocolate

Chips

Pizza

Biscuits

Cigarettes

Drugs

Candy!

Use charts as a guide, but don't worry too much if you find it difficult to memorize or if you have doubts whether your favorite food is alkaline enough. I, Elena, keep one of my 'alkaline charts' in my wallet at all times to reference at the grocery store!

FREE COMPLIMENTARY DOWNLOAD

We also have easy printable charts that you can download at no cost at www.bitly.com/alkalinecharts

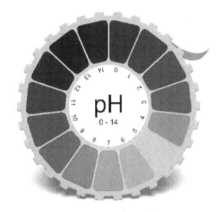

Problems with your download?

Email us at: elenajamesbooks@gmail.com

Now, that being said, or *read* rather, here are some ways to really boost the alkalinity of your diet!

1. Root vegetables are awesome!
   They are known for their healing power, you will find them used extensively in Chinese medicinal practices. They are also high in their mineral count. Turnip, beet, carrot, and rutabaga are all great examples of yummy alkaline root vegetables that will make your mouth water and are easily integrated into a variety of recipes (creative salads and soups).

2. The cruciferous variety will really enhance your alkalinity and your menu!
   They are full of vitamins and minerals. They add fiber and are downright tasty. Don't limit yourself to broccoli or cauliflower; forget not the cabbage or Brussels sprouts because they will add a unique flavor to many dishes. These are great steamed and then blended into creamy soups. We love to spice up our alkaline soups with a bit of chicken or fish. This is how we create our alkaline paleo mix and stick to the balanced alkaline rule of 70/30 (or even better 80/20- more on that at the end of this chapter).

3. <u>Do not leave out the leaves!</u>

   Leafy green vegetables are super alkalizing and can be added to or based around many recipes. Spinach, a variety of kale, Swiss chard, are my top three and are included in most of the meals that I eat in some way, shape or form. They are brimming with alkalizing essentials. Get committed to green, alkaline smoothies. If you can't stand the taste, or even the mere thought of having a green smoothie, simply blend in a banana, some coconut milk, cinnamon and nutmeg- so yummy and healthy, even kale can taste awesome, right?).

4. <u>Garlic is miraculous.</u>

   It is a detoxifying agent and is on many different health food lists. It will work as an antibiotic as well as being antifungal. It lowers blood-pressure and is a serious disease killer. Let us not forget how it easily adds flavor to an innumerable amount of dishes. Of course, nobody wants to overdose garlic (I guess we don't need to explain why?). We recommend you add half of a small garlic clove (minced) to your salad. It will make it taste delicious and help you detoxify, yet you won't experience bad breath. You can also mix ¼-1/2 garlic clove with your veggie smoothies and juices to give it more taste. We also go as far as using cumin and curry in our smoothies. We very often convert them into creamy soups. We just can't recommend coconut and almond milk enough. Both alkaline and paleo friendly!

5. <u>Cayenne pepper will add spice to your alkaline life.</u>
Capsicum is a super spice for alkalinity. It also works as an antibacterial agent in your system. Many people do not know that it contains vitamin A. You can add cayenne to many recipes (soups, juices, salads) or just drink mixed with water. We like to mix cayenne pepper with some olive oil and create our amazingly spicy dressing for salads. We also throw in some herbs like rosemary and thyme. These are both alkaline and paleo friendly.

6. <u>Limes and lemons are a great way to up the alkaline ante!</u>
They may seem acidic at first, because they taste acidic, but when they are processed by the body, they have an alkaline forming effect- this is what determines their alkalinity. They will stimulate your liver aiding in detoxification. They contain large amounts of vitamin C as well. Squeeze them into your water and add them to a variety of meals! Don't forget to serve your salads and

other meals like veggie stirs with a slice of lemon or a small glass of fresh lemon or lime juice. Grapefruits are also extremely alkaline. Oranges are more acidic but still healthy. If you want to have an orange juice, make sure you use fresh, organic lemons and mix it with a bit of alkaline water. High content of Vitamin C makes oranges alkaline, unfortunately they are also rich in sugars which makes them acidic. We love oranges and so do our kids, and we use them as a healthy treat. However, we have gotten used to lemons and grapefruits and we use these to detoxify and reach a healthy, alkaline balance in our lives.

Paleo: James' favorite part

Paleo is just my way of life and I have been following a balanced Paleo lifestyle (at least 90% Paleo) for more than 5 years now. Whenever asked if switching to Paleo was easy, I must admit that it wasn't. But the moment I began to see results, I fell in love with Paleo and it became my second nature. I really do believe that this diet was designed for carnivorous animals, like me!

The Paleo-way is a method of eating foods that our ancient ancestors would have foraged for, hunted and gathered. Why on earth, with all of the modern advancements and technology available, would we want to regress to eating like a caveperson? Well, with modern advancements have come modern problems.

The average diet today is full of health hazards. Obesity, disease, and digestive issues can all be traced back to the poor diet that is commonly ingested by the masses. These problems became prevalent after the agricultural revolution. So, the idea is that if we go back to a more simplistic, ancient way of eating, we can rid ourselves of the modern problems caused by contemporary developments in agriculture. There is no definite answer as to whether or not this is the reason why we are a fat, disease ridden population. Yet, we can see the benefit in going back to eating the things that we were biologically designed to process.

Grains and legumes (at least most of them), processed foods and oils, sugars and dairy are all foods that we began eating after the agricultural revolution. These are all items that we leave behind, following in our hunter-gatherer relatives' footsteps. Hey, at least you can go to the Farmer's market or grocery store instead of battling a saber toothed tiger on your way to pick up tonight's dinner.

My wife, Elena, drools over a huge bowl of salad. What tickles *my* salivary glands are large pieces of meat. I love meat. If there were better meat desserts I would be in heaven. She and I have never quite seen eye to eye on this issue, as she was always vegan and alkaline drawn, and I was a kid in a candy store at the butcher's counter. I do eat many vegetables as well. When I found the Paleo plan it just made sense to me and it was extremely easy to prepare. Chicken salad and tuna salad were always on my menu!

Ela jumped on the prehistoric bandwagon as well. She was very healthy as a vegan, but the lack of animal fats and protein was taking a toll on her. She was having problems with menopause. I had also noticed that she was having to put in long hours at work because she was having issues with thinking and concentration. We finally visited a naturopathic Chinese doctor and he examined Ela's case. He actually told her that her body will benefit from small portions of meat and fish. Since Ela is not big on red meat, we decided to add more fresh fish and seafood as well as organic chicken to her diet

Elena's health issues (as well as hair loss) began to fix themselves after we decided to try combining our nutritional perspectives. We were so ecstatic!

In our meeting of the minds, we realized that only a few things would need to be changed in order to Paleo-tize her alkaline lifestyle. In order to combine the two and yield the highest results, the 20% non-alkaline foods would now be focused on meat and eggs. We needed to negate all grains and grasses from her alkaline diet. Also tossed out the vegan window were all legumes and beans. Ahhhh no more soy makes me a happy Paleo boy! (of course, I allow her to have her strictly vegan style days, especially now that I know she is healthy). I believe that you can create your own diet and combine different dietary approaches. If soy and legumes work fine with your stomach, there is no need to follow this 100% strict Paleo band wagon. Listen to your body and give it what it needs.

So, in addition to the alkaline list, I am proud to present you with the Paleo list! Hey it may only be twenty percent, but I will take what I can get!!

- Organic, cage-free, free-range eggs
- Wild caught fish
- Lean cuts of grass-fed meat

**Rule of thumb: THERE SHOULD BE NO INDREDIENTS ON THE LABEL.

As a Paleo fan, I love the fact that you can eat typical lunches or dinners for breakfast. This helps me keep variety in my meals! An added bonus for sure.

It sounds overwhelming at first. When in actuality, it is very simple. If I can do it you can. I am a simple kind of guy. These Alkaline-Paleo guidelines were super easy for me to follow. Ela is a stickler for detail, I like a no-frills approach; once again this nutritional marriage proved itself to be a match made in heaven.

So, now that you know what you CAN eat (you understand the basic outline and allowable ingredients), let us move to the recipes. The recipes we have laid out for you all include meat (small amounts though); allowing us to showcase the Paleo-Alkaline twist.

Like we said in the description and the introduction, this book is about combining two different dietary approaches without becoming 100% alkaline zealot. We want balance, right?

Your everyday meal plan will also include meals without the meat/Paleo. Remember that the twenty percent consists of meat, so, if you have 3-5 meals in a day you only want a small percentage of each to be Paleo-laden. You can also consider having a larger portion meat in one or a couple of your meals and vegan alkaline meals for the rest of the day. Create whatever suits you and your lifestyle. If you are a fitness person, this alkaline paleo lifestyle will keep you energized and toned up.

Keeping your snacks and drinks strictly high alkaline will help too. Mix and match as you please, just be sure to stick to 80-70/20-30 as closely as you can!

One more thing- water! If you can't stand drinking pure water, we suggest you infuse it with fruits and herbs.

When having meat, make it 20% of your plate. The rest 80% should be alkaline veggies or other alkaline/Paleo friendly ingredients. This is really easy to do when you get used to salads and massive veggie stir fries that you can spice up with a bit of meat and fish.

Chapter 2 Alkaline Paleo Breakfasts to Start Your Day with a Bang

Breakfast can definitely be the most important meal of the day. The first meal sets the tone for what your body will be craving for the remainder of your waking hours. If you choose a Paleo-infused meal, you will get your proteins and healthy fats in right out of the gate! Begin your morning with one of these tasty Paleo-pumped recipes that are full of alkalinity as well. Aside from the actual recipes, we have also included our nutritional wellness tips so that you can create your own healthy dishes. It's really easy once you understand the rules of Paleo and Alkalinity.

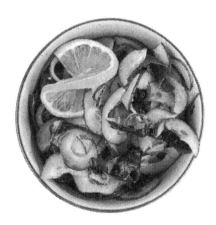

Recipe #1 Alkalinity Scramble

This tasty egg dish is quick to put together. Simple to prepare and mouth-watering! Our sons love it too!

Ingredients: serves 2

- 4 organic eggs

- 1-1 ½ cups spinach

- ½ cup sliced or chopped mushrooms

- ½ cup chopped onion

- 1 chopped or minced garlic clove

- 1 TBSP chopped basil

- ½ red bell pepper chopped

- ½ tsp salt

- 1 TBSP coconut oil

- ½ tsp cayenne (optional)

Preparation

1. Whisk the eggs in a bowl.

2. In a frying pan, heat oil to medium (or medium high) and then add pepper and onion. Cook for 2 minutes.

3. Add in the eggs, spinach, mushroom, garlic, and basil.

4. Cook and stir until eggs are done. Sprinkle with salt and cayenne.

Our tips:

You can also use olive oil if you wish. We are both great fans of coconut oil. There is no need to use acid-forming margarines and butters. Switch to good oils: coconut oil (also excellent in smoothies), avocado oil, and olive oil are our recommendations.

Craving sugar and sweets? Take 1 tablespoon of coconut oil. It will prevent the cravings. Try it- it really works. Coconut oil offers us good and healthy fats that we need to stimulate our metabolism. You can also experiment with herb and garlic infused oils. Organic olive oil (cold-pressed) is great for that. You can also use it in veggie smoothies to add to its nutritional value.

Recipe#2 Belly Breakfast

I, James, adore bacon. If bacon had asked for my hand in marriage, I would have had to seriously think about it (not too sure if Elena would like it though). This recipe will curb a craving for chemical-laden bacon, while providing healthy fats and alkaline veggies. You will not miss a thing! I love this breakfast before hitting the gym. It gives me all I need to successfully complete my workout!

Ingredients: serves 2

- ¼ lb. pork belly sliced thin or pancetta (ask the butcher to do it, tastes like bacon but healthier!)

- ½ onion diced

- ½ bell pepper diced

- 3 asparagus spears diced

- 1 ½ cups spinach

- 1 tablespoon coconut oil (may not be necessary depending

- ½ teaspoon nutmeg

- 1 teaspoon cumin

- 1 tablespoon diced cilantro

- 1 tablespoon diced parsley

- Pinch of salt

- 2 cups favorite salad greens (we use dandelion)

- Big squeeze of lemon juice for the salad greens

- 2 eggs

Preparation

1. Put egg and spices in a separate bowl and whisk well, set off to the side

2. Melt the coconut oil in a frying pan over medium. Fry up the pork. When it is cooked fully and browned, remove and allow to drain on paper towels. Leave the rest of the oil in the pan.

3. Add and sauté the asparagus for three minutes, then add the bell pepper and onion cooking for three more minutes.

4. Mix in the spinach, pork, and egg. Cook for 4-5 minutes, until the egg is set, flipping every so often.

Divide into two servings and top with cilantro/parsley. Serve with greens and add a squeeze of lemon.

Additional tips- make sure you add all kinds of spices and herbs to your shopping list. These are both alkaline and paleo friendly and will transform every dish you make. They will also provide you with a taste of variety. Our number one recipe for health and dieting success- spice it up as much as possible!

Do you need more Alkalinity? Have a glass of green juice first thing in the morning. It will wake you up- seriously! Green juices are now our "natural green caffeine". They also reduce food cravings and help you stick to your planned serves. They make you feel good and energized first thing in the morning and make the process of breakfast preparation a really nice ritual.

Many people don't like green juices and can't even stand the idea of drinking it on an empty stomach. We were there. It all comes down to getting used to it. Life is all about making choices. Sometimes we must do things that we don't really enjoy only to achieve higher goals. This is the reason many people go to work, right? So no more excuses, make sure you get your greens and do a 30 days "juicing in the morning" challenge. We are not talking about juice cleanse, this is our "healthy maintenance idea". You can have your balanced alkaline-paleo breakfast as always. But first...juice! You can thank us later.

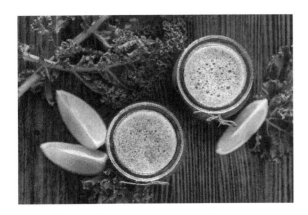

Simple recipe:

Juice 1 cup kale + 1 cup spinach + 1 apple to taste + half inch ginger + 1 lime + 2 carrots + 1 cucumber.

This recipe is great for weight loss and quick energy as you are feeding your body with zillions of nutrients!

Recipe#3 Salmon-y Sliders

We serve this breakfast anytime we have company. Everyone loves it. It is interesting and so yummy! It is my (Ela's) favorite as she loves fish of all kind. You can do as I do, and use it for a lunch as well!

Ingredients: serves 2

- 8 Portobello mushrooms (caps only)

- 4 eggs

- 4 ounces smoked salmon

- A few handfuls of spinach

- ½ each onion and cucumber thinly sliced

- Cayenne pepper to taste

- 2-3 Tablespoons coconut oil

Preparation

1. Using a large frying pan or skillet melt 2 tablespoons of coconut oil over medium heat. Add the mushroom caps, face down, and turn to medium low. Cook for 5 min. Remove and set on paper towels to drain.

2. Fry the eggs in the same pan over medium for five minutes or until set.

3. Set up your siders. Put one mushroom cap face up, then add the egg, a little salmon, and sprinkle with cayenne. Then add the spinach, onion and cucumber. Top with another cap face down.

You may find that one is enough, if you have a smaller appetite!

If you want to make it more alkaline, serve some tomato, carrot and bell pepper slices on side. Raw veggies are always good and a must for any alkaline-Paleo fan.

Recipe#4 Paleo-packed Peppers

This recipe will give you a vegetable kick start, while providing you with some of your Paleo for the day. These peppers are delectable! We had never contemplated using stuffed peppers for breakfast. Such a great way to start the day!

Ingredients: serves 2

- 2 bell peppers any color

- 4 organic free range eggs

- 1 c. mushrooms

- 1 c. broccoli florets

- ½ c. kale

- ½ teaspoon cayenne (omit if you do not like the spice)

- Salt/pepper (to your liking)

Preparation

1. Chop/dice your veggies (not peppers).

2. Set oven to 375 Fahrenheit (190 Celsius) and allow to preheat.

3. Whisk your eggs, seasoning, and vegetables in a bowl.

4. Carefully cut bell peppers in half (top to bottom), and remove stems and ribs/seeds.

5. Lay bell peppers on a cookie sheet, open side up, like a bowl. Use ¼ egg mixture in each. Add more vegetables if the mix does not fill it up all of the way.

6. Bake for 35 min or so, checking to make sure the eggs are cooked.

Recipe#5 Apple-Sausage Squash Salad

Nothing beats the smell of home cooked meals (James just said, "Except when you get to eat one!"). The aroma of this meal always has him sitting at the table, fork in hand, before it is even ready.

Ingredients: serves 4

- 1 lb. sliced chicken or pork sausage

- 1 green tart (granny smith) apple (chopped)

- 3 cups butternut squash chopped (if fresh cook it, or use frozen)

- 1 tsp garlic powder

- ½ tsp each cinnamon and nutmeg

- Enough spinach or leafy greens for a small plate of salad x4 (about 1 c. each)

Preparation

1. In a large frying pan brown the sausage and apple over medium. When the sausage is done, drain and set aside.

2. Put your squash in the pan and heat over medium low until warm. Sprinkle with the spices and stir in the sausage/apple mix.

3. Serve over salad. The simple one that we recommend when you are pressed for time, is a cup of spinach leaves with a few cucumber and tomato slices spiced up with a few drizzles of herb infused olive oil, if you can also add avocado slices, you will be hitting Alkalinity first thing in the morning and keep your stomach full and satisfied. There is no reason to be a martyr and live only on greens. Try our breakfast and enjoy the pleasure of balanced eating!

Recipe#6 Breakfast Bake

This next dish satiates my desire for a baked breakfast casserole. Just like mom used to make! It is full of alkaline vegetables and healthy eggs!

Ingredients: serves 4

- 1 tablespoon coconut oil

- ½ cup bell pepper (chopped)

- 1/2 cup onion (chopped)

- 1 cup spinach

- 2 cups kale (chopped and de-ribbed)

- ½ zucchini chopped

- 8 organic eggs

- 1/2 cup almond milk

- Salt/pepper/crushed red pepper (as much as you like)

Preparation

1. Set oven to 350 Fahrenheit (175 Celsius). Whisk eggs and milk in a bowl. Season with salt/peppers.

53

2. Heat a large cast iron skillet over medium with the coconut oil. Cook your onion and peppers for 3 min, the onion will be clear when it is ready.

3. Put in the kale and cook 5 min.

4. Add zucchini, spinach, and eggs, cooking 4 more min.

5. Now put in the oven to bake for 12-15 min. It must be cooked through.

6. Enjoy!

Recipe#7 Spicy Sweet Potatoes

I, Elena, make this dish every weekend! I love the spiciness combined with the sweet potatoes. I know you will love it too!

<u>Ingredients: serves 2</u>

- 2 sweet potatoes (cubed)

- 1 chopped onion

- 1 teaspoon cayenne

- 1 chopped, seeded jalapeno

- 1 bell pepper chopped and seeded

- ½ c. grape or cherry tomatoes chopped in half

- 2 TBSP chopped cilantro

- 2 tsp. cumin

- 2 eggs

- 2 TBSP coconut oil

Preparation

1. Heat coconut oil, medium heat, in a frying pan. Add the potatoes, jalapeno onions, and seasonings. Put a lid on it and cook until soft, about 5 min.

2. Take the lid off and allow it to brown for 3 min.

3. Put in all other ingredients, except the eggs. Allow to cook 3 more min, stirring constantly.

4. In the middle of the pan, use a spoon to make a crater in the middle and crack the eggs into it. Put the lid back on and cook three minutes longer (or until eggs look done).

Recipe#8 Berry Beefy

Ok, this is James' absolute favorite breakfast. The first time he made it, I had the "you have got to be kidding me" look on my face. He surprised me for sure, and you will be surprised as well. It is so tasty! To be honest, I am not a beef person but for this one, I will make an exception...

Ingredients: serves 4

- 1 lb. super lean ground beef

- 2 tablespoons coconut oil

- 4 cups blueberries

- Cinnamon to taste

Preparation

1. Heat a frying pan to medium with coconut oil. Add ground beef and brown till almost done. Sprinkle with a few shakes of cinnamon.

2. Turn off heat and mix in the blueberries. Keep in the pan and stir for 2 min.

3. Serve and enjoy!

Recipe #8 Yummy Shrimp Veggie Stir-Fry

Here comes another recipe that Elena loves. It's easy to digest and full of nutrients and healthy proteins. (James finds zucchini a bit boring, but thanks to yummy shrimps in this recipe, he got used to it).

Ingredients: serves 2

- 1 cup of shrimps (peeled and ready to eat)
- 1 garlic clove, minced
- 2 big zucchini, cubed into small pieces or sliced
- 1 red bell pepper, diced
- Pinch of Himalaya Salt
- Coconut oil
- 1 teaspoon of rosemary herb
- Pinch of curry and chili powder
- 1 cup of mushrooms

Preparation
1. Heat a frying pan to medium with coconut oil (about 2 tablespoons).

2. Add shrimps and then zucchini, ball pepper and mushrooms.

3. Stir fry adding some garlic, salt and spiced.

4. Make sure zucchini is nicely done-not too raw but also not too soft.

5. Serve and enjoy! We recommend you sprinkle over some lemon juice to make this recipe more alkaline.

Recipe#9 Simple Oregano Tuna Stir Fry

We love Italian spices. This recipe will help you love the alkaline-paleo diet first thing in the morning. Just try it yourself!

Ingredients: serves 2

- 2 cans of tuna
- 2 garlic cloves, minced
- 4 tomatoes, sliced and chopped
- 2 tablespoons of almond powder
- 1 tablespoon of fresh oregano
- 1 cup of mushrooms
- A few onion slices
- One small bell pepper, finely chopped
- Olive oil and Himalaya salt

Preparation
1. Heat a frying pan to medium with olive oil.
2. Add garlic and onion. Stir fry for a couple of minutes.
3. Then add mushrooms and bell pepper. Carry on stir frying for a few minutes until soft.
4. Now add tuna and mix well. Add oregano and keep stir frying. You may add a bit more of olive oil.

5. Spice up with some oregano and almond powder. You will feel like eating pizza again!

The key to success is transforming the dishes you love into new, healthy ones. We oftentimes crave pizza and pasta because we want flavors. Simply stir-fry some veggies with oregano and almond powder or other powdered nuts and give yourself this amazing healthy alkaline paleo pleasure.

*****

We very often let our bodies rest from animal protein. It's easy for me (Elena) but a bit of a challenge for James, he loves his meat. However, I very often tell him that our Paleolithic ancestors also had no-meat periods. They were not only hunters, but also gatherers, right? I never get it why so many Paleo people stuff themselves with meat. Not long ago, I realized that I want to help Paleo people find healthy, alkaline balance and follow the Paleolithic philosophy at the same time. Don't be afraid to become a gatherer!

Recipe#10 Vegan Paleo Breakfast

We love this simple raw breakfast in the summer. We usually spend summers in the South of Spain and it can be really, really hot there.

Ingredients: serves 2

- Half cup of almonds
- One cup of blueberries (these are full of antioxidants)
- One apple, cut into slices
- 1 banana, sliced
- Half cup of dried fruits of your choice (make sure they're sugar free)
- 2 cups of almond milk and a bit of coconut milk or cream for the top
- Cinnamon to spice up
- OPTIONAL: 1 teaspoon of organic spirulina or chlorella powder
    Preparation
    Simply mix all the ingredients in a bowl.

Almond milk and coconut milk are both alkaline and Paleo. This breakfast is moderately alkaline and will keep your stomach full. We also love it when we crave something sweet. Fruit is a natural, healthy treat to fall back on.

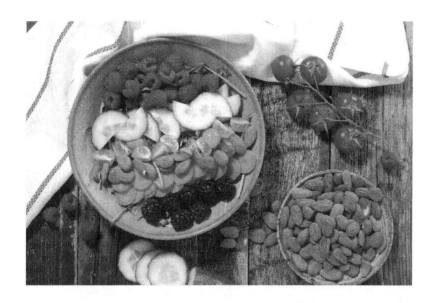

Chapter 3: Lasting Lunches: Alkaline with a Splash of Paleo

For some, lunch is a pain; you have to stop your momentum in getting things done to fuel the body and mind. For others, it is a welcomed break in the day. Either way, these Alkaline-Paleo lunches will make your stomach full and your mouth happy!

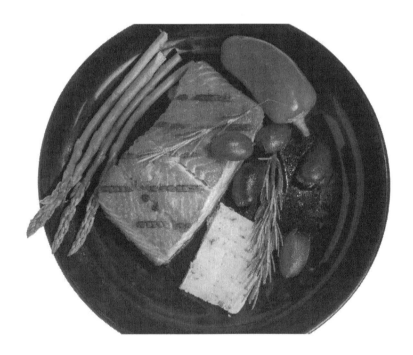

Recipe#11 Salmon Salad Sandwiches with Simple Salad on the Side

We were big fans of tuna salad sandwiches. This recipe allowed us to rid our fridge of mayonnaise and still curb the craving. It replaces bread with sweet potato slices!

Ingredients: serves 2-3

- 1 lb. salmon fillet=1.5 cups salmon for your salad
- salt/pepper to taste
- ½ lemon's juice
- ½ lemon's zest
- 1 stalk of celery, chop well
- 1.5 teaspoons dill, fresh chop well
- 1 tablespoon extra-virgin olive oil
- Small handful of baby spinach for each sandwich

Preparation

1. Season salmon. Bake in a preheated oven, 350 Fahrenheit (157 Celsius) for about 10 min. It will be flaky when done.
2. Put in a mixing bowl.
3. Add in the all other ingredients and mix well with a fork.

65

Recipe#12 Sweet Potato Bread

- 1 large sweet potato (Works better with short wide ones as opposed to long/skinny) sliced ¼ inch thick
- 4 TBSP coconut oil
- ¼ tsp each: paprika and cumin
- 1 tsp garlic powder
- 1 pinch of salt

1. Heat oven (450 Fahrenheit or: 230 Celsius)).
2. Put a wire rack on a baking sheet.
3. In a bowl, mix the spices up with a fork.
4. Using a large bowl or a large zip lock bag, coat the sweet potato in the coconut oil. Add the spices and coat well. Put on the rack.
5. Bake for 35-40 min. Top with more salt if you like.

Now to assemble your sandwiches! Take one piece of "bread" and put a large scoop of salmon salad on it. Top with spinach and another slice of "bread." Serve with salad below!

Recipe#13 Simple Salad

<u>Ingredients</u>

- 1 bunch kale, torn

- ¼ cup raw almonds, chopped

- Half of an avocado, chopped

- 3 tbsp. coconut oil, melted

- Pinch of cayenne

- Pinch of sea salt

- Juice of half a lemon

- Fresh pepper

1. Mix salt, cayenne, oil, lemon, and pepper in a small bowl with a fork.

2. Toss the avocado and kale with the dressing and serve with sandwiches.

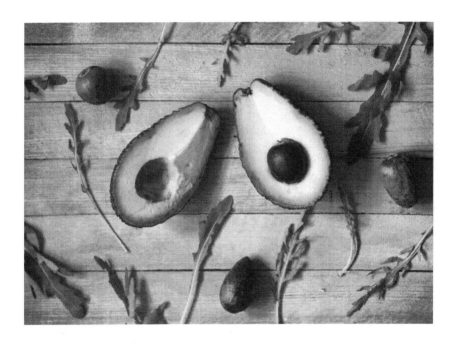

Recipe#14 Carne Asada with Kale Chips n' Spinach Guacamole

We adore Mexican food! We love nachos and carne asada. This is our go to meal anytime we want some south of the border flavor.

Ingredients: serves 2-4

Crockpot Carne:

- Approx. 2 lb. lean chuck roast

- 1 orange and 2 limes juiced

- ¼ cup evoo

- ½ cup chopped cilantro

- 2 tsp crushed red pepper

- 5 crushed, chopped or minced garlic cloves

- 2 tsp oregano

- ½ tsp cumin

- 4 green onion bulbs chopped or 1 shallot

- 1 teaspoon sea salt

Preparation

1. Rinse your beef and trim all visible fat. Allow to dry ½ hour.

2. Put the other ingredients in food processor. Simply pulse for a min.

3. Put in crockpot. Coat the meat, rubbing it with the marinade.

4. Put about 1/3 cup of water in the bottom of your crockpot.

5. Cook on high for about 5 hours. Slice across grain.

Serve slices on 2 stacked kale chips, dolloped with guac.

Recipe#15 Guac

- 2 avocados (peeled and pitted)

- 1 large lime (juice)

- 1 cucumber

- 8 c. spinach chopped

- ½ c. cilantro chopped

- ½ cup chopped onion

- 1 tsp. cumin

1. Put all, except cucumber and onion, into blender/processor and mix well. Stir the chopped cucumber and onion into the mix by hand.

2. Put in the fridge.

Recipe#16 Kale Chips

- 2 bunches of kale

- 3-4 tablespoons olive oil

- Salt (as much as you like)

- Cayenne (if you want them spicy)

1. Preheat the oven to 300 Fahrenheit (150 Celsius). Remove the rib by slicing top to bottom on each side of it. Then cut each side in half if they are long. If they are short then leave whole (you want to put the carne on top so the leaves will be longer than normal kale chips). 3-4 inches each will work.

2. Wash and dry the leaves, drying is very important: use paper towels or clean towels if needed.

3. I then put the kale, half at a time, in a large bowl or zip lock. Then put in half the oil with each batch, massaging with hands to coat.

4. Lay out on baking sheets and do not overlap. Season.

5. Put sheets in the oven and bake until crispy. Normally I rotate the trays after about 5 min. They usually take 3 min. longer. Do not allow them to brown. They taste

nasty! When they are crisp, remove from oven. Transfer onto to paper towels to cool.

Now use two stacked on top of each other, put a thin slice of carne and some guac on top. Do not place the meat on the chip until you are going to put it in your mouth. I usually serve the meat and guac on plates and then give each person a separate serving of chips.

******

Recipe#17 Soup n' Souper-Salad

Soup and salad is a classic way to eat lunch. This chicken soup is delicious. It is mild in flavor and will balance the addictive tangy, flavor-packed salad.

Ingredients: serves 2

Prepare salad first (at least a few hours ahead)

Souper-salad:

- 1/2 head cabbage (red) shred

- 1 ½ cups kale (chopped)

- ½ red onion (slice thin)

- ½ cup radishes sliced

- ½ sliced cucumber

- 1 cup raw (not pasteurized) sauerkraut

- 2 sliced green onions

- 3 tbsp chopped mint

- 3 tbsp coconut oil

- 2 tbsp apple cider vinegar

- 1 tbsp maple syrup

- 2 teaspoons Dijon mustard

- ½ tsp cayenne

Preparation

1. Put all of the veggies in a bowl.

2. Whisk together the ingredients for the dressing in another bowl.

3. Add the dressing and stir to combine. Allow to set a few hours.

Serve with soup!

Recipe#18 Soup

- 1 quart chicken broth

- ½ lb. shredded cooked chicken (leftovers work well)

- 1 large rib celery, dice or chop

- 1 large carrot, dice or chop

- 1 zucchini, use a grater, peeler or slicer to make noodles

- Salt/pepper to taste (if you like crushed red pepper or cayenne please add)

1. Boil the broth and add the cooked chicken. Turn to low and simmer

2. Put in the carrots and celery for 20 min.

3. Now, add noodles and cook 3-4 min longer.

Recipe#19 Chicken-Strip Salad

James misses breaded chicken sometimes. Breading in almond meal is a Paleo-acceptable way to prepare chicken. He loves these strips a-top my favorite salad!

Ingredients: serves 2-3

- 1 pound chicken breast (boneless and skinless)

- 1 cup almond meal

- 1 heaping tablespoon paprika

- 1 teaspoon garlic powder

- 1 teaspoon cayenne pepper

- 1 teaspoon coarse ground pepper

- 1 teaspoon salt

- 2 eggs (beat)

- A few tablespoons oil to grease baking sheets

  Preparation

1. Heat your oven (375 Fahrenheit or 190 Celsius)).

2. Cut your chicken into one or two inch wide strips.

3. Mix the meal and spices.

4. Grease baking sheets.

5. Dunk each piece of chicken in the egg and then roll in the meal.

6. Put the chicken on baking sheets in the oven for 25 min or so until crispy and brown.

Make salad and then serve chicken on the salad.

Recipe#20 Salad

- 1 lb. baby spinach

- ½ of a lemon (to squeeze)

- ¼ cup coconut oil

- A few splashes of coconut aminos (your preference)

- 1 large avocado, dice

- ¼ cup chopped almonds

1. Wash and dry spinach.

2. Mix all dressing ingredients in bowl and stir in the avocado.

3. Now combine all of the ingredients toss well.

Recipe#21 Asian Meatballs with Noodles

This meatball recipe will fill your kitchen with delicious Far East aromas! The noodles are made of zucchini; bring on the alkalinity!

Ingredients: serves 4

Noodle Salad

- 1 large extra-large zucchini

- 2 tablespoons rice vinegar

- 1 teaspoon sesame oil

- ¼ teaspoon red pepper flakes

- ½ teaspoon coconut aminos

- ½ teaspoon ginger powder

- Salt/pepper

1. Take a carrot peeler, peel up your entire zucchini up into noodles. Stir in all of your other ingredients as well. Allow flavors to combine for at least twenty minutes while you prepare the meatball.

Paleo Meatballs

- 2 lbs pork (ground)
- 2 teaspoons salt
- 1 teaspoon coriander
- ½ teaspoon white pepper (use black if you want)
- ½ teaspoon cayenne
- 2 tsp crushed red pepper
- 2 teaspoons fish sauce
- 1 tablespoon sesame oil
- 2 Tablespoons coconut aminos
- 1 ½ piece of ginger, grated
- 1/3 cup cilantro (chop)
- 4 scallion bulbs (chop)

1. Mix the pork, salt, coriander, peppers, fish sauce, oil, aminos, ginger, cilantro and scallion in a bowl. Sprinkle spices all around, do not dump them in.

2. Squish up with your hands to combine all well. Do not squish meat too much or it may toughen when cooked.

3. Cover two cookie sheets with parchment paper: one for cooking and one for cooling. Roll the meatballs (they should be about a tablespoon).

4. Use a large skillet and heat to medium high. Add your meatballs. You will have to make a few batches because they need room in order to brown.

5. They will cook for a total of about twenty minutes. Turn them three times during the cooking process. Transfer to the other baking sheets. Until they are all done.

Recipe#22 Simple Vegan Paleo Salad

We love seaweed like kombu or wakame. These are both alkaline and Paleo friendly and we recommend you start using them in your salads. Like we have already mentioned before, it's good to do a few days without meat every now and then. This recipe should give you some ideas as for vegan Paleo options. It's all about healthy variety, right?

Ingredients (serves 2)

- A few square inches of wakame
- A few square inches of kombu
- One cup of radish
- 2 avocados, sliced and pitted
- Half cup of almonds
- 2 tablespoons of chia seeds
- ¼ cup raisins (raisins and onion are an excellent taste combination!)
- Half onion, minced
- 2 big tomatoes
- Olive oil
- Juice of 1 lemon
- Himalaya salt

OPTIONAL: if you really need some animal protein, add tuna or raw shrimps /salmon

Preparation

1. Soak wakame and kombu in water (you may want to slice it first) for about 10m mins.
2. In the meantime, mix other ingredients in a big bowl.
3. Add olive oil and lemon juice.
4. Finally, mixed in wakame and kombu.
5. Enjoy, we do!

Chapter 4 Delectable Alkaline Dinners

Ending the day on a good note is important in our home, as I am sure it is in yours. Choosing to eat your meaty meal at the end of the day can be a welcomed treat, especially if you are like James and need motivation in the form of meat to push you through.

This dinner recipe sounds funny but tastes delicious. Bison adds a great flavor to these balls. The alkaline roasted vegetables compliment the flavor well!

Recipe#23 Bison Balls and Roast Veggies

Ingredients: serves 4-6

- 2 pounds ground bison (you can use whatever lean ground meat you like)
- 1/2 an onion, chop
- 1 ½ teaspoons sea salt
- 1 teaspoon cumin
- ½ teaspoon cayenne
- ½ teaspoon black pepper
- 2 cups spinach, chop and pack tightly
- ½ cup cilantro
- 2 beaten eggs

Preparation

1. Set oven to 400 Fahrenheit (200 Celsius). Cover baking sheets with parchment paper.
2. Mix everything in a bowl with hands.
3. Roll into balls, about 1 heaping tablespoon of mix per ball.
4. Bake 25 min. They need to be browning and cooked through.

Recipe#24 Roast Veggies

- 1 head cauliflower, chop
- 1 squash (which ever you like), peel and cube
- 2 chopped beets
- 1 large zucchini
- 2 large carrots
- 2 tablespoons coconut oil
- 2 tablespoons fresh parsley, chop
- 1 teaspoon cayenne
- 1 tablespoon black pepper
- 1 tablespoon rosemary

Preparation

1. Set oven to 400 Fahrenheit (200 Celsius).
2. Mix all veggies in a bowl, but keep zucchini separate. Toss the mixed veggies with most of the oil save a little bit.
3. Spread the vegetables out on a cookie sheet and sprinkle with salt and pepper.
4. Roast for 20 min.
5. Coat zucchini and season with salt/pepper.
6. Add zucchini to the other vegetables and stir, roasting ten more min.
7. Sprinkle with rosemary and parsley.

Recipe#25 Barbeque Chicken and Coleslaw

This dinner is great for summer! Even in the dead of winter it is delicious and will help you to have a taste of July in January! We love this coleslaw and receive nothing but compliments on it.

Ingredients: serves 2-4

- 1 chicken (whole, guts removed)
- 1 onion, slice
- 3 teaspoons paprika
- 1 teaspoon sea salt
- 1 teaspoon onion powder
- 1 teaspoon thyme
- 1 teaspoon white pepper
- 1 teaspoon cayenne
- 5 minced garlic cloves
- 1 teaspoon black pepper

Preparation

1. Dry chicken thoroughly.
2. Put onions in the bottom of the crockpot.
3. Put the chicken on the onions.

4. Mix all of the ingredients in another bowl. This will be your rub, using your hands massage the chicken with the seasonings (outside and inside).

5. Cook set to low setting for at least six hours or until done.

Recipe#26 Coleslaw

- 2 cups green cabbage, shred
- 2 cups red cabbage, shred
- 2 bell peppers sliced thin
- 4 carrots, julienned
- 2 cups bok choy
- 3 tablespoons chives chopped
- 2 tablespoons coconut aminos
- 2 tablespoons coconut oil
- ½ lemon to squeeze for juice
- 1 tablespoon sesame oil
- 3 teaspoons freshly grated ginger root
- 2 teaspoons tahini
- Pinch of sea salt

Preparation

1. Mix all of the veggies in a bowl. In another bowl whisk your dressing ingredients. Pour over vegetables and coat well. Serve it as soon as you toss it!

Recipe#27 Italian Beef

I, Ela, had an Italian grandmother and I miss her cooking oh so much. When I make this recipe, my kitchen smells like grandma's did, so many years ago. I have taken out the pasta and replaced it with my favorite: zucchini noodles (I cannot get enough of these).

Ingredients: serves 2-4

- 4 lb. round roast

- Few tablespoons of oil (olive or coconut)

- 2 onions, slice

- 5 cloves garlic, minced

- 2 teaspoons garlic powder

- 2 tablespoons oregano divided in half

- 3 c. raw baby carrots

Preparation

1. Sear the roast on both sides in a dutch-oven, using high heat. Make sure that it browns well on both sides before flipping. Add some oil, turn down to medium high, and brown on all sides for a few minutes. Take out the roast and set aside.

2. Turn the heat even lower, to medium. Put in both garlic and onion. Cook for three or four minutes.

3. Sprinkle the meat with oregano and garlic powder, then put back in the pan.

4. Pour in a cup of cold water, put the lid on and simmer over medium low for three and a half hours or so. If you need, add a bit more water. I might check every hour. After two hours, put in the baby carrots, sprinkle with the rest of the garlic powder and oregano.

5. When done, take out the meat and slice. Serve over noodles below with carrots on the side.

Recipe#28 Zucchini Noodles

- 2 medium zucchinis

- 1 cup baby spinach per serving

- 1 tablespoon olive oil

- 1 garlic clove, minced

- Salt/pepper

1. Use a box style grater using the big holes. Chop off the tips of the zucchini.

2. Push along the grater with pushing the length of the zucchini, making long noodles.

3. Use a pan and heat the oil to medium. Fry the noodles for a few minutes until tender.

Place spinach on the plate, then a serving of noodles, and finally the beef and carrots.

Recipe#29 Topped Tilapia with Kale Salad

We adore tilapia. It is replaceable with other white fish in this recipe. I sometimes make a double recipe of the pesto, as it is a favorite in our home and very versatile!

Ingredients (serves 2)

- 4 tilapia filets

- 1 tablespoon olive oil

- 2 cloves garlic

- 2 tablespoons water

- 30 basil leaves

- 1 inch chunk of zucchini (peel)

  Preparation

1. Blend in food processor or blender all but tilapia in blender, taa daah pesto sauce.

2. Spread over tilapia.

3. Allow oven to preheat to 400 Fahrenheit (200 Celsius)

4. Bake for 20 minutes.

Recipe#30 Krispy Kale Salad

- 2 bunches kale, stems removed and torn
- 1 c. fennel, chop
- 10 baby radishes, shred
- 2 tablespoons olive oil
- Pinch of sea salt
- Big squeeze of lemon

Mix well in a bowl, serve alongside tilapia.

When you want some comfort food and do not want to fall off the wagon, prepare this recipe. The fried chicken and mashed potatoes included are Alkaline-Paleo, but will kill the urge to cheat!

Recipe#31 Chicken, Sprouts, n Spuds

<u>Ingredients: serves 2</u>

Chicken and Sprouts

- 2 chicken leg quarters
- ¼ c. veggie broth
- 1 stalk of Brussels Sprouts (remove stem)
- 1 ½ tablespoon coconut oil
- Salt, black and crushed red pepper to taste
- 3 crushed garlic cloves
- 1 tablespoon olive oil
- 1 lemon to squeeze

<u>Preparation</u>

1. Allow oven to heat to 425 Fahrenheit (220 Celsius)
2. Prepare your sprouts, and then half them.
3. Coat the sprouts in olive oil. Sprinkle with salt/peppers.
4. Season rinsed and dried chicken as well.
5. Put coconut oil in a cast iron skillet and heat over medium to medium-high.
6. When heated, put in the chicken, skin side down. Allow to cook until nice and crunchy. 5-8 min. Do not move them around in the pan.

7. When this is done, flip and do the same for the underside.
8. Add sprouts, ¼ c. broth, and squeeze the lemon in. Mix well.
9. Bake in oven for half of an hour, or until chicken is done.

Recipe#32 Spuds

- 6 sweet potatoes
- 1 ½ cups coconut milk
- 1 tablespoon coconut oil
- 1 tablespoon salt
- 1 teaspoon pepper
- 1 tsp cayenne
- 1 ½ teaspoons curry

1. Chop the potatoes and boil for 18-22 minutes.
2. When soft, drain then mash them, mixing in the other ingredients.

Serve alongside chicken and Brussels.

BONUS CHAPTER: Alkaline Paleo Salads

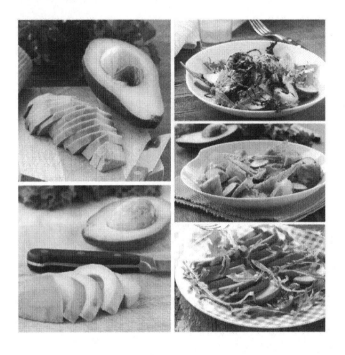

Recipe#32 Apple and Celery Root Salad

Servings: 2-3

Ingredients

- 1 medium red apple, skin-on and diced
- 2 tablespoons of crashed cashew nuts mixed with 2 tablespoons of coconut oil (our vegan mayo!)
- 1 tablespoon of Dijon Mustard (to our knowledge- this is Paleo acceptable)
- 1 medium sized celery root, peeled and grated
- 4 tablespoons of chopped walnuts
- Paleo Gremolade(1 tablespoon)
- Juice of 1 lemon
- 2 scallions (sliced)
- Half cup of thick coconut yogurt
- Half cup of minced fresh parsley leaves

Method of preparation

1. Toss celery root with diced apples and lemon juice. Then add-in the scallions, walnuts and parsley. Toss again to combine.
2. Mix the gremolade and mayonnaise with coconut yoghurt in another bowl.

3. Add the mayonnaise salad dressing to the apples mixture and then toss to combine.
4. Cover the salad bowl with saran wrap and refrigerate for at least 2-3 hours before serving.

Recipe#33 Samphire Roast Lemon and Hazelnut Salad

Servings: 2-3

Ingredients:

- oz. (180 grams) of Samphire
- Organic maple syrup(1-2 tablespoons)
- 0.881 oz. (25 grams) of hazelnuts
- 1 whole lemon, sliced
- 3 whole radishes
- Olive oil (about 2 tablespoons)

Ingredients for the dressing:

- Paleo maple syrup (1 tablespoon)
- Olive Oil (2 tablespoons)
- Fresh juice of half a lemon
- 2 tablespoons of finely chopped fresh mint leaves

Method of preparation:

1. Preheat an oven to 446 degrees Fahrenheit (230 Celsius). Slice lemon into thin slices.
2. Combine the olive oil and maple syrup in a bowl. Dip

the lemon slices in the maple syrup mixture and transfer to a parchment paper lined baking tray.

3. Insert the tray in the oven and roast for 15-20 mins until the lemon slices start to brown.

4. Mix olive oil with maple syrup and lemon juice in a bowl. Whisk well to combine and then add-in the mint leaves to prepare the dressing.

5. Lay the hazelnuts in a baking tray and roast in the oven for 5 minutes.

6. Steam the samphire for 1 minute over a steamer in the meantime and then rinse the leaves under cold water. Drain properly and set aside.

7. Finally, toss the steamed samphire leaves with the roasted lemon slices and hazelnuts. Drizzle the seasoning on top and toss again to serve.

Recipe#34 Green Papaya Salad

Servings: 2

<u>Ingredients</u>

- oz. (50g) of mixed fresh lettuce leaves
- ½ of a green papaya, julienned
- 1 whole radish, sliced
- ½ of a small carrot, julienned
- 2 tablespoons of raw cashew nuts
- 2-3 whole cherry tomatoes, quartered

<u>For the Chilli Dressing</u>

- Coconut vinegar (1 tablespoon)
- Raw honey (1 tablespoon)
- 2 tablespoons of water
- 1 red long chili,(remove the seeds and chop)
- A bit of of fresh lime juice
- 1 tablespoon of Paleo fish sauce
- 1 small clove of garlic, peeled and minced

Method of preparation

1. Toss the julienned carrots and papaya with radish and lettuce leaves. Place in a bowl. Top with the quartered cherry tomatoes and cashews. Set aside.
2. In a separate bowl take the chili slices and add the other ingredients required for the dressing. Whisk to combine.
3. Drizzle the dressing over the salad and serve with lemon wedges.

Recipe#35 Summer Slaw with Tahini Coconut Dressing

Servings: 4

Ingredients for slaw

- 1 head of fennel, cored and sliced
- 1/4th cup of raisins
- 1/4th of a head of purple cabbage, cored and sliced
- Half cup of Thai basil
- 1 bell pepper /remove seeds and slice/

Ingredients for the dressing

- 1 tablespoon of coconut milk
- 2 tablespoons of paleo tahini
- 1-inch of fresh ginger, grated
- 1 teaspoon of paleo raw honey
- Lime juice (use 1 lime)
- 1 teaspoon of sea salt
- Black pepper, to taste

Ingredients for curried cashews

- 1 cup of raw cashew nuts
- 1/4th teaspoon of paprika

- 1 tablespoon of raw coconut oil
- 1 tablespoon of lime juice
- 1 ½ teaspoons of paleo curry powder
- 1/4th teaspoon of chili powder
- 1/4th teaspoon of turmeric powder

Method of preparation

1. To prepare the cashews, heat up 1-2 tablespoons of organic coconut oil in a pan and add the lemon juice and herbs to the oil. Stir for a minute and then drop the cashews in the oil.
2. Stir the nuts in the oil for a minute and transfer to a parchment paper lined cookie sheet.
3. Bake the nuts in a 350 degrees Fahrenheit (or 175 Celsius) preheated oven for 10-15 minutes. Remove once done and let cool.
4. To prepare the slaw, toss the chopped fennel with cabbage, basil leaves and yellow pepper slices.
5. Whisk all the dressing ingredients until a smooth dressing is formed.
6. Drizzle the dressing over the slaw and drop the raisins and cashew nuts on top to serve.

Recipe#36 Raw Broccoli Slaw

Ingredients

- 1 cup of carrots(shredded)
- ½ cup of fresh red cherries
- 1½ cups of broccoli florets, shredded
- 3/4th cup of red cabbage, shredded
- ½ cup of thinly sliced red onion
- 1 cup of baby kale leaves

Dressing

- 3 teaspoons of chia seeds
- 4 teaspoon of paleo Dijon mustard
- 6 tablespoon of coconut vinegar
- 6 tablespoons of extra virgin olive oil
- 1/4th cup of raw honey
- 1/4th teaspoon of black pepper
- ½ teaspoon of kosher salt

Method of preparation

1. Process the carrots and broccoli florets in a food processor to shred those. Place in a large bowl. Add the

onion slices, cherries, kale leaves and shredded red cabbage.

2. Prepare the dressing by mixing everything in a separate bowl.

3. Drizzle the dressing over the slaw and toss before serving.

It can also be serve as a broccoli cream.

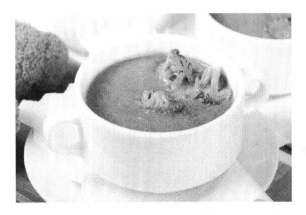

Don't forget to pick up your FREE GIFT...

Free Complimentary eBook

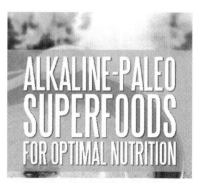

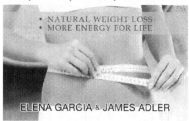

Download link:

www.bitly.com/alkapaleofree

Problems with your download?

Contact us: elenajamesbooks@gmail.com

Conclusion: Take Positive Action Today!

We provided a basic rundown of the Alkaline and Paleolithic lifestyles. You now have food lists and recipes. The only thing left to do is to start preparing these meals and change your life for the better!

You will notice improvements in all areas. Your brain will flourish! You will have tons of energy, lose weight, and health issues will improve quickly. No longer will you need to implement and search for cures and quick fixes. The answer is in changing your dietary habits!

Vegetable lovers can have their "cake" and eat it too! Meat fanatics will be allowed a nice portion of mouthwatering animal goodness while still alkalizing their bodies! You will love the balance incorporated in this nutritional lifestyle. You will LOVE the results that you will indefinitely see and experience.

By living according to an Alkaline-Paleo blueprint, you are essentially giving your body the fuel it was designed to run on.

111

You will be feeding yourself and your family the foods that your body needs in order to function optimally! Do not waste another day! Get started now, feel the health benefits immediately! Life is short; enjoy it to the fullest by eating Alkaline-Paleo based foods.

To your success,

Elena and James

PS. If you enjoyed this book, please take the time to share your thoughts and post a review on Amazon. It would be greatly appreciated! Your comments are very important to us.

Follow us at:

www.facebook.com/HolisticWellnessBooks

www.twitter.com/WellnessBooks

FREE AUDIOBOOK FROM HOLISTIC WELLNESS BOOKS

If you would like to lose weight or transform your body we have an amazing free resource that can help you on your journey.

It's a mindset-changing free audio program called: "NLP for Fast Weight Loss". Its kindle and paperback versions have been very popular on Amazon and hit the bestsellers' ranks in motivational reads. We are now giving you the audio version for free. You can listen to it while driving, cleaning or...cooking your healthy Paleo-Alkaline meals!

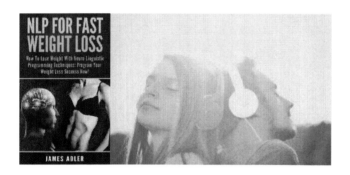

Grab your free copy from:

www.bitly.com/freehwaudio

Recommended Reading

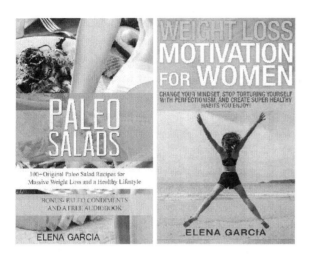

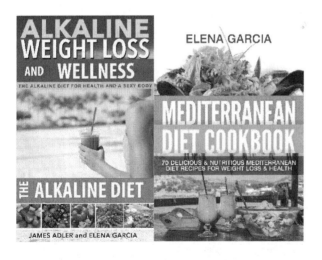

Available in all Amazon stores (kindle and paperback formats)

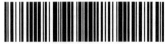

Made in the USA
Middletown, DE
26 August 2016